JUICING FOR IDEAL HEALTH

Delicious And Essential Guide To Healing Common Disease, Increase Energy, Weight Loss And Staying Healthy For Life.

EPIPHANY HUB PRINTS

JUICING FOR IDEAL HEALTH

COPYRIGHT © 2023 BY EPIPHANY HUB PRINTS

TABLE OF CONTENT

LAUNCH INTO AN EXTRAORDINARY JOURNEY OF DISCOVERY AND ENLIGHTENMENT AS YOU DELVE INTO THE PAGES OF THIS CAPTIVATING BOOK, WHERE EACH CHAPTER UNFOLDS LIKE A TREASURE WAITING TO BE UNEARTHED, PROMISING TO IGNITE YOUR IMAGINATION, TEST YOUR BELIEFS, AND LEAVE AN INDELIBLE MARK ON YOUR HEART AND MIND.

IN OUR BOOK SHELF WE'VE ALREADY CREATED

"THE ULTIMATE LOW CARB DIET RECIPES COOKBOOK FOR BEGINNERS"

HERE IS THE LINK …PLEASE CLICK!

"DIABETES BREAKFAST RECIPES MEAL PLAN FOR WOMEN"

HERE IS THE LINK….PLEASE CLICK

"COMPLETE MEDITERRANEAN RECIPES COOKBOOK FOR SENIORS"

HERE IS THE LINK….PLEASE CLICK

"KIDNEY RECIPES FOR THE NEWLY DIAGNOSED"

HERE IS THE LINK….PLEASE CLICK

INTRODUCTION

Seeking good health is more important than ever in a society when life seems to be moving at an ever-increasing pace. It's a journey that frequently takes us down many different pathways, but the transforming potential of juicing is one that has drawn a lot of attention. Allow me to take you on a tour of the colorful world of juicing, where the combination of tastes tantalizes the senses and feeds the body from the inside out.

Imagine a busy metropolis where people are trying to manage job, family, and personal well-being and the daily grind is taking a toll on them. Among them is Emily, a dynamic professional who enjoys life but is experiencing wear and tear from a demanding way of living. In the process of trying to live a better lifestyle, she discovered the wonderful world of juicing.

It all began with a simple realization: the secret to opening a reservoir of vitality was hidden in the vivid hues of fruits and vegetables. Captivated, Emily set out to investigate the art of juicing, armed with a blender and a selection of fresh produce. As she set out on this adventure, she learned the secret to transforming the abundance of nature into delectable concoctions that not only delighted her palate but also revitalize her entire being.

Her palate was transformed by the rainbow of fruits and vegetables, and each mixture conveyed a message of wellbeing. Each component contributed to this symphony of flavors and nutrients, including the vivid greens of spinach and kale, the fiery reds of strawberries and beets, and the sunny yellows of mangoes and citrus fruits.

Emily saw a significant change in her skin tone, energy levels, and general vitality as she continued to juice. The combination of vitamins, minerals, and antioxidants from the freshly squeezed juices formed a powerful concoction that strengthened her defenses against illness and gave her a natural supply of long-lasting vitality.

We discover the significant influence that juicing can have on our pursuit of optimal health via Emily's experience. Come along as we examine the science and art of juicing and see how this straightforward yet effective habit can serve as a stepping stone to a happier, healthier existence. Juicing is a transforming lifestyle that encourages us to sip our way to vitality; it's more than simply a fad.

CHAPTER ONE: INTRODUCTION TO JUICING

Understanding the Basics of Juicing

Juicing is a way of eating that provides a concentrated and readily absorbed version of vital nutrients by drawing the liquid out of fruits, vegetables, and herbs. Juicing is usually done with a juicer to separate the juice from the pulp, resulting in a cool drink that is rich in enzymes, vitamins, minerals, and antioxidants.

Benefits of Including Juicing in Your Diet

Enhanced Absorption of Nutrients: Juicing presents a practical approach to ingest an assortment of fruits and vegetables, offering a concentrated supply of vital nutrients. Due to dietary restrictions, people with renal illness frequently struggle to satisfy their nutritional needs, thus this can be especially helpful to them.

Support for Hydration: A lot of fruits and vegetables are high in water, which helps with hydration. Maintaining proper hydration is essential for kidney health since it aids in the body's removal of waste and toxins. For those who may find it difficult to drink ordinary water, juicing might be a great approach to increase fluid intake.

Simple Digestion: By removing the fiber from the liquid during the juice extraction process, the body is better able to absorb nutrients. Because it lessens the strain on the digestive system and could lower the stress on impaired kidneys, this can be beneficial for those who have kidney disease.

Packed with Antioxidants: Antioxidants are found in a lot of fruits and vegetables and are very important in keeping the body's damaging free radicals in check. Controlling oxidative stress is essential for those with kidney disease, and an antioxidant-rich diet can improve general health.

Variety and Flavor: Juicing makes it possible to eat a variety of fruits and vegetables in a fun and varied way. This type not only tastes better, but it also guarantees a wider range of nutrients, which supports general health and energy.

How Juicing Supports Overall Health in Relation to Kidney Health

Managed Nutrient Intake: Juicing offers a planned and regulated approach to consume vital nutrients while adhering to certain dietary restrictions that are frequently connected to renal illness. This makes it easier for people to get the nutrition they need without consuming too much potassium and phosphorus, which can damage the kidneys.

Personalization for Renal-Friendly Diets: Juicing enables the development of recipes that are specially suited to the requirements of people who have renal disease. For example, adding low-phosphorus and low-potassium fruits and vegetables guarantees a kidney-friendly drink that complies with dietary recommendations.

Support for Hydration Goals: It's important to maintain an appropriate fluid balance because kidney function and hydration are strongly related. Juicing can help achieve hydration objectives by providing a tasty substitute for plain water and preventing excessive fluid consumption, which may be prohibited in some situations.

Reduction of Digestive Difficulties: Digestive problems are occasionally linked to kidney illness. Juicing offers a liquid version of nutrition that is easier on the digestive system, which may help those with digestive issues feel less uncomfortable.

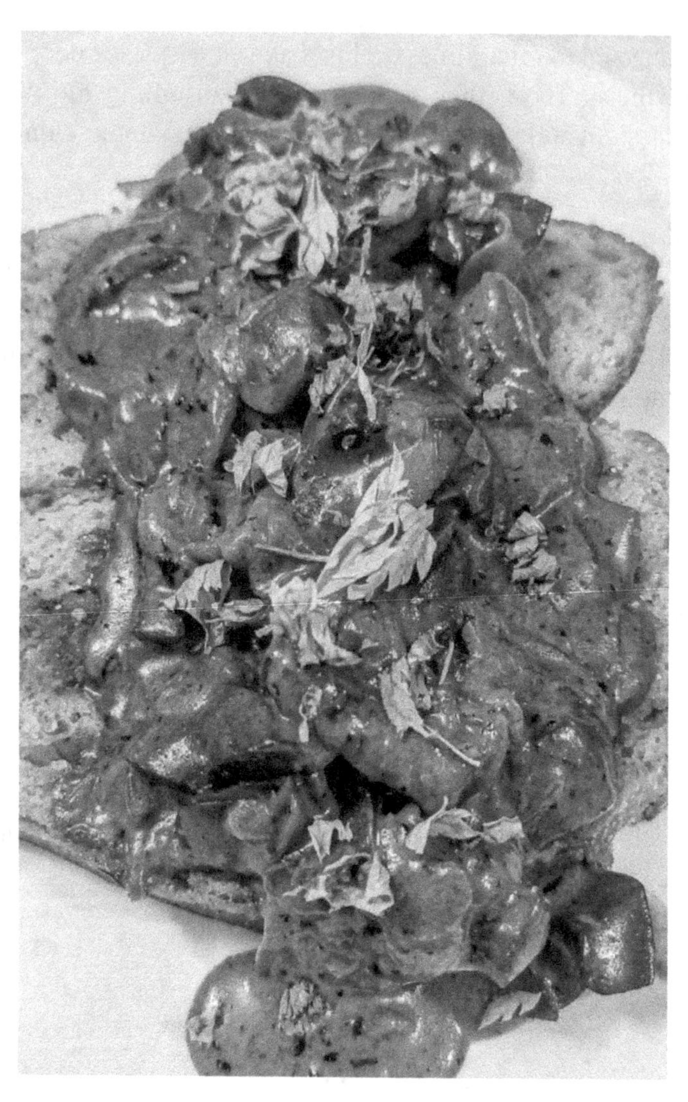

CHAPTER TWO

SELECTING THE RIGHT INGREDIENTS

Choosing Nutrient-Rich Fruits and Vegetables for Kidney-Friendly Juicing

When juicing to support kidney health, it's important to use fruits and vegetables that are high in nutrients. Making the appropriate decisions can improve your juices' nutritional profile by adding vital vitamins and minerals without sacrificing kidney function.

Berries: Antioxidant-rich and low in potassium, berries like blueberries, strawberries, and raspberries are great options for kidney-friendly juicing.

Apples: Apples naturally sweeten drinks without adding a lot of sugar, and they are low in potassium. To lessen the fiber content, make sure to peel them.

Cucumbers: Rich in water and low in potassium, cucumbers help you stay hydrated and give your juices a cool flavor.

Watermelon: A fruit that helps maintain fluid balance and provides flavor, watermelon is hydrating and has a low potassium content.

Carrots: Carrots naturally sweeten your juices and are a rich source of beta-carotene. They are kidney-friendly since they often contain less potassium.

Embracing Seasonal and Organic Options:

Seasonal Variety: To get the most out of freshness and flavor, use seasonal fruits and vegetables. Seasonal produce may spice up your juicing routine and is frequently more economical.

Selecting Organic Produce: To reduce your exposure to artificial chemicals and pesticides, think about selecting organic produce. Even while it's crucial to wash fruits and vegetables, choosing organic produce could provide you with extra piece of mind, particularly if you want to use the skin or peel in your juices.

Balancing Flavors for Optimal Taste and Nutrition:

Balance of Sweet and sour: To create a well-rounded flavor profile, combine sweet fruits, like apples, with sour ones, like berries. This guarantees a well-rounded nutritious intake in addition to satisfying the palate.

Add Greens: Leafy greens that don't drastically affect potassium levels, including kale, spinach, or Swiss chard, can give your juices an extra nutritional boost. They also help create a flavor profile that is more harmonious.

Herbs and Spices: To improve the flavor of your kidney-friendly juices, try experimenting with herbs like mint or spices like ginger. These can offer a burst of flavor without using too much sugar or salt.

Considerations for Kidney Health:

Monitoring Potassium: Although a lot of fruits and vegetables are good for your kidneys, it's important to keep an eye on your potassium levels, particularly if you have any dietary limitations. To find out how much potassium you specifically need, speak with a doctor or nutritionist.

Limit Foods High in Oxalate: Kidney stone production may be facilitated by the oxalates found in certain fruits and leafy greens. If you have a history of kidney stones, talk to your doctor about reducing the amount of oxalate-containing foods in your diet.

Fluid Intake: To promote kidney function, make sure you're getting enough water in addition to juicing. While juices help you stay hydrated, water is still the most important part of a kidney-friendly diet.

CHAPTER THREE
ESSENTIAL EQUIPMENT AND TECHNIQUES

Overview of Juicers and Blenders for Kidney-Friendly Juicing

Blenders and juicers are useful appliances for adding nutrient-dense liquids to a diet that is healthy to the kidneys. Comprehending their characteristics and appropriate utilization is essential for optimizing nutritional advantages while taking into account the dietary limitations linked to renal well-being.

1. Juicers: Extracting Nutrients Efficiently

The purpose of juicers is to extract liquid from fruits and vegetables while sifting out the tough pulp. Masticating and centrifugal are the two primary varieties.

Centrifugal Juicers:

Pros: Quick and effective, ideal for tough fruits and veggies.

Cons: Could produce heat, which could change the amount of nutrients.

Ideal for those who must restrict their consumption of fiber or potassium with regard to kidney function.

Masticating Juicers:

Pros: Best for soft fruits and leafy greens, as it preserves more nutrients when operating at slower speeds.

Cons: Slower than juicers using centrifugal force.

Kidney Concern: Great for preserving nutritional integrity, particularly in those with certain dietary needs.

2. Blenders: Retaining Fiber and Nutrients in Smoothies

In contrast, blenders combine all ingredients into a smoother texture while preserving fiber. There are several varieties available, such as personal blenders and high-speed blenders.

Fast-moving Blenders:

Pros: Smoothly blend fruits and veggies with fiber.

Cons: Possibly holds onto more fiber than centrifugal juicers.

Kidney Consideration: Good for people whose diets would benefit from more fiber.

Individual Blenders:

Pros: Encourages portion control and is convenient for single servings.

Cons: Not as huge as other blenders in terms of capacity.

Kidney Consideration: Suitable for people with particular dietary demands and portion sizes.

The Best Juicing Methods for Kidney-Friendly Diets to Get the Most Nutrition

Mix Up the Ingredients:

Include Variety: To guarantee a varied nutrient profile, include a variety of fruits and vegetables.

Potassium Sensitivity: Choose low-potassium foods and limit your intake of high-potassium foods.

Control Sugar Content:

Natural Sugars: Prefer fruits with natural sugars over those that have been added.

Harmonious Mixtures: Mix fruits and vegetables to maintain a balanced sugar content.

Control Your Sodium Intake:

Select Fresh Ingredients: Steer clear of processed or canned foods and instead choose fresh produce.

Herbs and Spices: To enhance taste without increasing salt content, use herbs and spices.

Experiment with Nutrient-Rich Additions:

Include Superfoods: Include kidney-friendly superfoods such as citrus fruits, berries, and leafy greens.

Balanced Macros: Try to have a good balance of fats, carbs, and proteins.

How to Keep Your Juicing Equipment Clean and Maintain It for Kidney-Friendly Hygiene

Quick Cleaning Following Usage:

Avoid Bacterial Growth: Juicers and blenders should be cleaned and rinsed right away to prevent the growth of bacteria.

Dismantle Parts that can be removed for thorough cleaning should be disassembled.

Use Mild Cleaning Agents:

Steer Clear of Harsh Chemicals: To avoid residual contamination, use natural cleaning solutions like vinegar or lemon.

Regular Maintenance: To guarantee peak performance, give your juicers a deep cleaning every few months.

Regularly check and replace parts:

Check Blades and Filters: Examine the blades and filters for wear and tear. Replace any clogged or dull filters as necessary.

Make Sure Tight Seals: To stop leaks, make sure rubber seals are tight on a regular basis.

Equipment Storage Done Right:

Dry Completely: Before storing, let every component air dry entirely.

Ventilation: To stop the growth of mold, store in an area with good ventilation.

CHAPTER FOUR

TAILORING JUICING TO YOUR HEALTH GOALS

Knowing How to Manage Your Weight in Relation to Your Kidney Health

Importance of Maintaining a Healthy Weight: The Value of Retaining a Healthy Weight Juicing provides a nutrient-dense, low-calorie alternative to excess weight, which can aggravate renal strain.

Balancing Nutrient Intake: Juicing provides for exact control over calorie and nutrient consumption, which supports weight management objectives.

Including Foods High in Nutrients but Low in Calories

Verdant Greens: Rich in nutrients, low in calories, and appropriate for people with kidney disease.

Low-Sugar Fruits: For sweetness without a lot of calories, go for melons and berries.

Optimizing the Macronutrient Content of Juices to Manage Weight

Addition of Protein: To improve satiety, add protein-rich items such as nut butter or Greek yogurt.

Healthy Fats: To add a pleasing texture and longer-lasting energy release, add avocados or flaxseeds.

Portion Control and Meal Replacement

Sensible Portions: Juicing can help you control your portion sizes and avoid overindulging.

Strategies for Meal Replacements: When done properly, switching from a meal to a balanced juice can help with weight management.

Boosting Energy and Vitality through Kidney-Friendly Juicing

Choosing Energizing Ingredients

Citrus Fruits: **High in vitamin C, promoting energy production and supporting the immune system.**

Beets and Carrots: **Rich in natural sugars and antioxidants, providing sustained energy.**

Incorporating Hydration and Electrolytes

Celery and Cucumber: **High water content helps stay hydrated without adding extra calories.**

Coconut Water: **A natural electrolyte supply that boosts energy levels.**

Avoiding Excessive Sugars for Sustainable Energy

Careful Fruit Selection: **To prevent energy surges and crashes, choose fruits with a lower natural sugar content.**

Bringing the Sweet and Savory Together: **To create a well-rounded flavor profile, mix sweet fruits and veggies.**

Addressing Specific Health Concerns Through Kidney-Friendly Juicing

Managing Blood Pressure

Beet juice: Nitrates found in beet juice have the potential to reduce blood pressure.

Potassium Considerations: To help with blood pressure management, select fruits and vegetables that are low in potassium.

Reducing Inflammation

Infusions of ginger and turmeric: Their anti-inflammatory qualities may be advantageous for kidney function.

Papaya and pineapple: These fruits' enzymes may help to lessen inflammation.

Supporting Kidney Function

Hydration Importance: Juices with a high water content are important for renal function generally and contribute to hydration.

Antioxidant-Rich Foods: Leafy greens and berries are rich sources of antioxidants that promote kidney health.

Catering to Dietary Restrictions

Low-Potassium Options: To comply with kidney diet guidelines, select fruits and vegetables that are lower in potassium.

Consultation with Medical Specialists: Always consult a dietician or healthcare professional to make sure juicing is appropriate for your particular health needs.

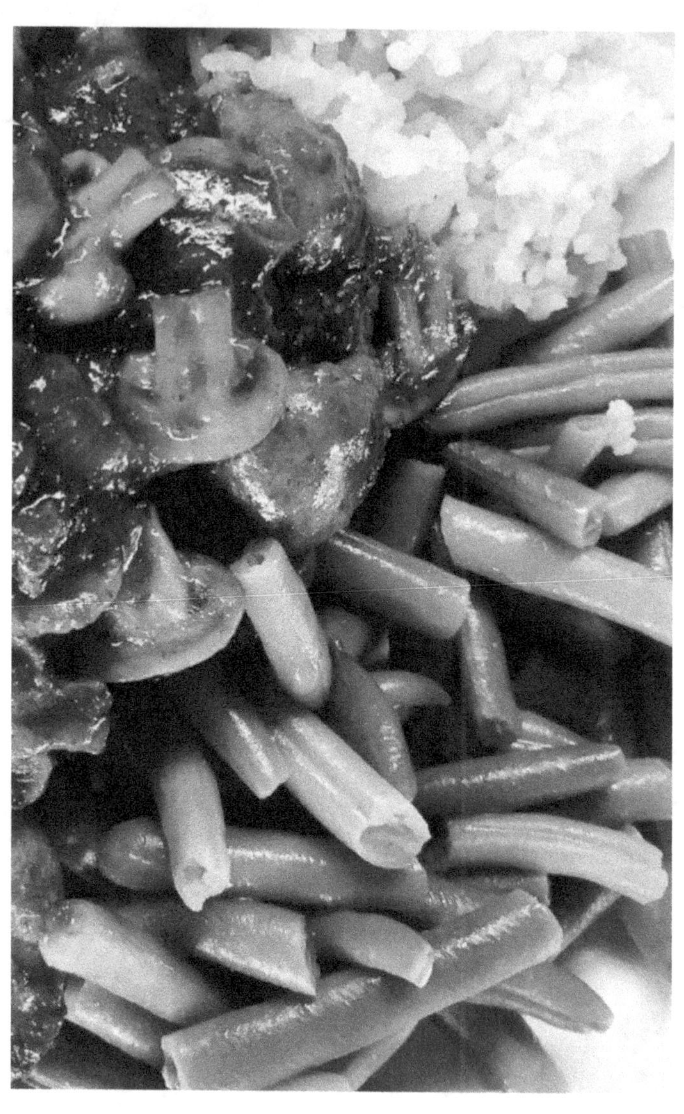

CHAPTER FIVE

CREATING NUTRIENT-PACKED RECIPES

Green Juices for Detoxification in the Context of Kidney Health

Green juices, with their abundance of nutrients and possible detoxifying effects, can be a great complement to a kidney-friendly diet. Detoxification must be approached carefully, though, particularly for those who have renal illness.

Incorporating Kidney-Safe Greens

Low-Potassium Greens: Opt for low-potassium greens such as cucumber, spinach, and kale.

Reducing Oxalates: To lessen the risk of kidney stone formation, be aware of the oxalate content and choose greens with lower oxalate concentration.

Detoxification Benefits

Support for Hydration: Green drinks help you stay hydrated generally, which is important for healthy kidney function.

Rich in Chlorophyll: By promoting liver function, chlorophyll, which is present in leafy greens, may help with detoxification.

Caution with High-Potassium Ingredients

Avocado moderating: Though rich in nutrients, avocados contain a lot of potassium, so limit your intake when using them in green drinks.

Ingredients for Balancing: To keep things in balance, mix low-potassium greens with other veggies that are good for kidneys.

Antioxidant-Rich Fruit Blends for Kidney Health

Antioxidant-rich fruits offer a tasty method to boost general well-being while adhering to dietary limitations, with several benefits for kidney health.

Selecting Fruits Safe for Kidneys

Berries: Rich in antioxidants and low in potassium are blueberries, strawberries, and raspberries.

Citrus Fruits: Grapefruits and oranges offer a flavorful and vitamin C-rich boost without being overly potassium-rich.

Antioxidant Benefits

Protecting Kidney Cells: By assisting in the neutralization of free radicals, antioxidants may be able to prevent damage to kidney cells.

Anti-Inflammatory Properties: Some fruits may help kidney health by having anti-inflammatory properties.

Conscientious Sugar Control

Natural Sugars: Avoid fruits with added or processed sugars and stick to those with natural sugars.

Juggling Sweet and Savory: To control the amount of sugar, mix sweet fruits with non-sweet veggies.

Balancing Macronutrients in Your Juices for Kidney Health

Achieving a balanced nutrient profile in your juices is essential for individuals with kidney disease, considering protein, carbohydrates, and fats.

Protein Considerations

Including Low-Phosphorus Proteins: Take note of your phosphorus levels and include sources such as hemp protein or almond milk.

Portion Control: To prevent overtaxing the kidneys, limit the amount of protein in juices.

Management of Carbohydrates

Selecting Complex Carbs: For long-lasting energy, choose fruits and vegetables that are high in complex carbs.

Fiber-Dense Supplements: Add high-fiber foods to promote the health of your digestive system.

Healthy Fats for Nutrient Absorption

Including Nutrient-Dense Fats: Chia seeds and avocados are good sources of healthy fats that aid in the absorption of nutrients.

Moderation is key: watch portion sizes to avoid consuming too many calories even though they are healthful.

CHAPTER SIX

INCORPORATING JUICING INTO YOUR DAILY ROUTINE

Breakfast Juices for a Healthy Start in the Context of Kidney Health

Energizing Citrus Blend

Ingredients: Grapefruits,

Oranges,

Plus a tiny bit of strawberries.

Benefits: Low in potassium and high in antioxidants and vitamin C.

Considering the Kidneys: Citrus fruits offer a cool beginning without consuming too much potassium.

Kidney-Cleansing Green Juice

Ingredients:

Cucumber,

Celery,

Kale, and

Dash of lemon juice are the ingredients.

Benefits: low in potassium and detoxifying qualities of cucumber.

Considering the Kidneys: Nutrient-rich greens and hydrating cucumbers support kidney function.

Low-Potassium Berry Blast

Ingredients: 1 tiny apple,

3 raspberries, and blueberries.

Benefits: High in antioxidants; moderate in potassium and natural carbohydrates.

Consideration for Kidneys: Provides a tasty choice without going above potassium thresholds.

Midday Energy Boosters and Snacks to Maintain Healthy Kidneys

Nut-Based Protein-Packed Smoothie

Ingredients: Banana,

Low-phosphorus protein powder, and

Almond milk.

Benefits: Phosphorus content should be considered; balanced protein for healthy muscles.

Consideration for the Kidneys: Supplies necessary amino acids without overloading the kidneys with phosphorus.

Refreshing Cucumber Mint Cooler

Ingredients:

Cucumber,

Mint leaves, and

Hint of ginger.

Benefits: Hydrating and low in potassium; aids digestion.

Consideration for Kidneys: Supports hydration without contributing to potassium overload.

Fiber-Rich Apple Carrot Delight

Ingredients: Apples,

Carrots, and

Dash of chia seeds are the ingredients.

Benefits: Moderate potassium content and high fiber content for digestive health.

Considering the Kidneys: Maintains nutritional balance and encourages regular bowel motions.

Evening Elixirs for Relaxation and Better Sleep with Kidney Health in Mind

Calming Chamomile Lavender Infusion

Ingredients:

Lavender,

Tiny bit of honey, and

Foundation of chamomile tea.

Benefits: Promotes better sleep by calming the neurological system.

Consideration for Kidneys: Low-impact substances that hydrate without taxing the kidneys are taken into consideration.

Golden Milk with Turmeric

Ingredients:

Almond milk,

Cinnamon,

Turmeric, and

Dash of black pepper

Benefits: Promotes kidney and joint health; has anti-inflammatory qualities.

 Considering the Kidneys: includes spices that are good for the kidneys and encourages relaxation.

Beetroot and Berry Sleep Tonic

Ingredients:

Mixed berries,

Beetroot juice, and

Spritz of coconut water.

Benefits: Berries provide antioxidants; beetroot promotes blood flow.

Thought for the Kidneys: Offers nourishment without too much potassium, encouraging a good night's sleep.

These carefully chosen recipes for juices and elixirs are meant to boost your diet's nutritional content while keeping renal health in mind. As always, for individualized guidance based on your unique health needs and dietary limitations, speak with a medical practitioner or a certified dietitian.

CHAPTER SEVEN

POTENTIAL CHALLENGES AND SOLUTIONS

Dealing with Sugar Content in Juices:

Even juices made from real fruits can include high levels of sugar, which can lead to health problems like blood sugar spikes and weight gain. Take into account the following tactics to lessen this:

Balance with Vegetables: To reduce total sugar level and increase vital nutrients, add a range of vegetables to your juices. Cucumbers, celery, and leafy greens are great options.

Select Low-Glycemic Fruits: To reduce the effect on blood sugar levels, choose fruits like berries and citrus that have lower glycemic indexes.

Water or Ice Diluting: You can lower the amount of sugar in each serving of your juice while still being properly hydrated by diluting it with water or adding ice cubes.

Investigate Herbal Infusions: You may reduce the amount of added sugar in your juices while adding new flavors by enhancing the flavor with herbal infusions like mint or basil.

Adapting Juicing for Dietary constraints:

Juicing remains beneficial for people who have particular dietary constraints, such as lactose intolerance or gluten intolerance.

Consider these tips:

Select Non-Allergenic Ingredients: Go for produce that is less likely to cause allergies or sensitivities, such as fruits, vegetables, and herbs. Nuts and several fruits are common sources of allergies, so watch what you choose.

Investigate Alternative Bases: To accommodate particular dietary requirements, try substituting coconut water, almond milk, or even green tea for conventional fruit juices.

Speak with a Nutritionist: If you have any dietary limitations, speaking with a nutritionist will assist you in developing customized juicing recipes that will meet your requirements for nutrients without containing any additives that could cause issues.

Sustainable Juicing Practices for Long-Term Health:

Juicing for health benefits shouldn't come at the price of the environment. Adopt sustainable habits to improve both your health and the health of the environment:

Select Locally produced Produce: When selecting seasonal fruits and vegetables for your juices, choose locally produced produce to help local farmers and lessen your carbon impact.

Employ Reusable Containers: To reduce the amount of single-use plastic waste related to store-bought juices, make an investment in reusable glass or stainless steel containers.

Compost Leftover Pulp: To cut down on kitchen waste and improve soil health, think about composting the leftover pulp from juicing instead of throwing it away.

Consumption with Mindfulness: Juice mindfully by only making what you need. This guarantees that you drink fresh, nutrient-rich juices and lessens food waste.

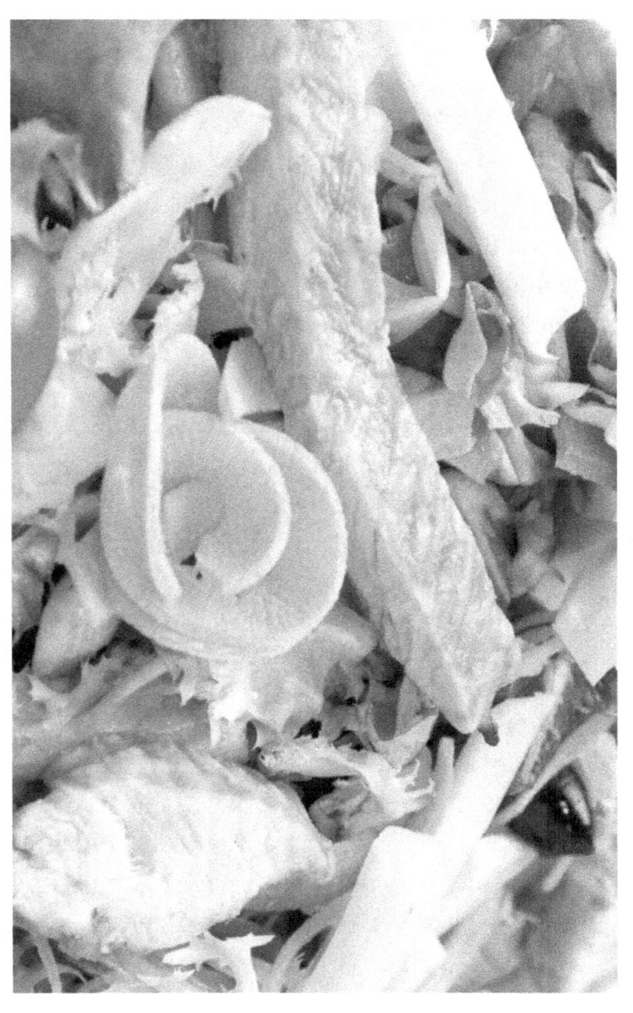

CONCLUSION

Small, deliberate decisions have a big role in the road toward good health in the colorful fabric of life. That is the story of juicing, a vibrant page in the book of health. The pulsating sound of the juicer serves as the transformation's background music as our main character sets off on his or her journey to find vitality.

Every mouthful of recently extracted nectar, according to this story, is a communion with nature's abundance—a symphony of nutrients dancing in a rainbow of flavors. With a rainbow-hued assortment of fruits and veggies and an apron stained with kale, our story's hero learns the alchemy of transforming simple, healthful components into liquid gold.

The protagonist experiences a plethora of health benefits in addition to an increase in vitality via the lens of juicing. Once-overlooked vegetables like kale, spinach, and beets become unsung heroes, adding antioxidants, vitamins, and minerals to the voyage. The pages turn, immunity strengthens, our hero's complexion brightens, and they get newfound energy that drives them onward.

In the epilogue, juicing is portrayed as a ray of health and a symbol of the wonder that occurs when we align with the natural color spectrum. The story's obvious lesson is that, in the larger scheme of wellbeing, juicing is a chapter that will never fade—a colorful, tasty monument to the ability to choose health, one drink at a time.